Nursing Professional and Practice Contexts

Quick and easy to reference, this short, clinically focused guide is ideal for use on placements or for revision.

The professional role of the nurse is at the very foundation of good care management and provision. Nurses are accountable to patients, the public, employers and their entire profession. It is imperative that you have a sound understanding of the various ethical, legal and professional issues you will face during your career. This competency-based text covers:

- Professional issues and accountability
- Communication
- The patient journey
- Diagnostic testing
- Care planning
- Managing and leading in the clinical environment
- End-of-life care

Outlining relevant key concepts, lifespan matters, assessment and nursing skills, it also helps you learn by including learning outcomes, concept map summaries, activities, questions and scenarios with sample answers, and critical reflection thinking points. It is suitable for pre-registration nurses, students on the nursing associate programme and newly qualified nurses.

Tina Moore is a Senior Lecturer in Adult Nursing at Middlesex University, UK. She teaches nursing assessment, clinical skills and acute care interventions for both pre-qualifying and post-qualifying nurses. Her interests are in simulated learning approaches and Objective Structured Clinical Examination (OSCE) as a teaching and assessment method. She has authored a number of books and articles. She is also a Middlesex University Teaching Fellow.

Sheila Cunningham is an Associate Professor in Adult Nursing at Middlesex University, UK. She has a breadth of experience teaching nurses both pre- and post-registration and she supports mentors supporting students in practice. She is also a Middlesex University Teaching Fellow and holds a Principal Fellowship at the Higher Education Academy. She is currently programme leader for the BSc European nursing.

Skills in Nursing Practice

Series editors
Tina Moore, *Middlesex University, UK*
Sheila Cunningham, *Middlesex University, UK*

This series of competency-based pocket guides covers relevant key concepts, anatomy and physiology, lifespan matters, assessment and nursing skills for good clinical practice in a range of areas from safety and protection to promoting homeostasis. To support your learning, they include learning outcomes, concept map summaries, activities, questions and scenarios with sample answers, and critical reflection thinking points.

Quick and easy to reference, these short skills-focused texts are ideal for use on placements or for revision. They are ideal for pre-registration nurses, students on the nursing associate programme and newly qualified nurses feeling in need of a little revision.

List of titles

Nursing Skills in Professional and Practice Contexts
Tina Moore and Sheila Cunningham

Nursing Skills in Safety and Protection
Sheila Cunningham and Tina Moore

Nursing Skills in Nutrition, Hydration and Elimination
Sheila Cunningham and Tina Moore

For more information about this series, please visit: www.routledge.com/Skills-in-Nursing-Practice/book-series/SNP

Nursing Skills in Professional and Practice Contexts

**Tina Moore and
Sheila Cunningham**

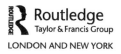
Routledge
Taylor & Francis Group

LONDON AND NEW YORK

First published 2020
by Routledge
2 Park Square, Milton Park, Abingdon, Oxon OX14 4RN

and by Routledge
52 Vanderbilt Avenue, New York, NY 10017

Routledge is an imprint of the Taylor & Francis Group, an informa business

British Library Cataloguing-in-Publication Data
A catalogue record for this book is available from the
British Library

Library of Congress Cataloging-in-Publication Data
A catalog record has been requested for this book

ISBN: 978-1-138-47948-7 hbk)
ISBN: 978-1-138-47949-4 (pbk)
ISBN: 978-1-351-06562-7 (ebk)

Typeset in Stone Serif
by Wearset Ltd, Boldon, Tyne and Wear

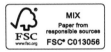

Printed and bound in Great Britain by
TJ International Ltd, Padstow, Cornwall

Contents

Figures

Introduction to the Skills in Nursing Practice series

This particular book is one in a series of six 'Nursing Skills in ...'.

Book 1 *Professional and Practice Context*
Book 2 *Protection and Safety*
Book 3 *Nutrition, Hydration and Elimination*
Book 4 *Control and Coordination*
Book 5 *Cardiorespiratory Assessment and Monitoring*
Book 6 *Mobility and Support*

These books are designed to be used in clinical practice and can be used not only for reference but also as an invaluable revision tool. There is a continuing emphasis on skills acquisition and development particularly within nursing. This is accompanied by the increasing understanding of the necessity to effectively and efficiently integrate theory and clinical skill competence-based learning. In doing so, it ensures that nurses have the best opportunity to become 'fit to practise' and develop key employability skills. Therefore, each chapter has been linked to the *Future Nurse Proficiencies* (Nursing and Midwifery Council [NMC] 2018a), which will enable you, as the reader, to map your skills development in relation to the standards set by the professional body.

The structure of each chapter within the books draws on the constructivist pedagogical approaches and assimilation theory. Each chapter has interlinking ideas and information through the use of concept maps. It is anticipated that the use of key words and connections will deepen and enhance these linkages from the concepts, drawing on general and specific aspects of a topic and will therefore promote active learning.

Concept maps are pictures or graphic representations that will help you to organise and represent knowledge of a subject.

This is achieved through helping you to link, differentiate and relate concepts to each other. The concept maps begin with a main idea (or concept) and then branch out to show how that main idea can be broken down into specific topics. They can also visually represent relationships between concepts and ideas in a quick, easy-to-understand format. Concept mapping is becoming increasingly popular as a means of teaching and learning within education. The introduction of concept maps will provide a quick summary **with** additional key information of the material read in the *Clinical Skills for Nursing Practice* book. We have also included related anatomy and physiology together with life span matters.

The end of each chapter has questions (answers also provided) in the format of a quiz. This will help you to test your knowledge, understanding and application of the content. There is also the opportunity for you to critically reflect on your learning using a SMART (specific, measureable, achievable, realistic and time-frame) format. From this you should then be able to clearly identify areas for future development and learning.

These pocket-size books are designed not only to help develop further your clinical skills (practice and knowledge), but also to improve your key transferrable skills, enabling them to advance your employability skills, i.e. problem solving, analytical and critical thinking, and team working. Therefore another aim for each book is to concentrate on scaffolding learning, as a result supporting, promoting and developing autonomous learning, questioning and critical thinking. The use of concept mapping allows reorganisation of information in a visual manner to promote critical thinking in the student nurse. Through concept mapping students can see how ideas/patient care needs and the interrelationships that exist promote critical thinking in relation to clinical practice.

The books within this series are not designed to be comprehensive text books. It is the practice companion of the *Clinical Skills for Nursing Practice*, and is designed to be used together with that book. The design of these 'pocket-size' books will enable students/readers to use them as a resource while working within and outside of in clinical practice.

Tina Moore and Sheila Cunningham

Introduction and overview

Working within a professional discipline, there are boundaries of professional standards and regulations. A number of key policies were published just before and after the investigation and publication of the final Francis report in January 2013 (Francis 2013; Keogh 2013). This report detailed the serious failings at the Mid Staffordshire NHS Foundation Trust and poor leadership, in particular, has been highlighted as one of the main reasons for the organisational failures that led to this and a number of other high-profile incidents. The Francis report details 290 recommendations for improvements in care, culture and education. Twenty-nine of these recommendations specifically focused on nursing. This report and the subsequent dissection and analysis by the media, professionals and policy makers are considered as being a watershed moment for nursing.

To be a professional is to be engaged in activities that are guided by a body of knowledge and evidence. Nurses need to feel confident and proud of their profession, and strive further to make positive contributions to multidisciplinary care in an ever-changing and politically driven healthcare arena. Along with this are the legal and professional influences/implications in relation to professional accountability. It is important that student nurses aiming to gain entry to the register have an understanding of why all nurses are bound by a professional code of conduct and what constitutes the hallmarks of professional behaviour as dictated by the Nursing and Midwifery Council (NMC 2018b). In addition to practising in accordance with the 'The Code' and as a reflective practitioner, nurses also need to consider their own values, beliefs and actions in terms of how this translates into professionalism.

Communication is one of the fundamental roles of a nurse. The nurse's ability to communicate effectively will be put to the test throughout their career in nursing. This is because nursing involves working with a wide range of people across the life-span, within a multicultural society and when people are at their most vulnerable. Even during one shift a nurse will experience different styles, different styles of communication, different influences on the communication transactions and changes in communication when a person is ill.

Feeling vulnerable can lead people to behave in ways that may be challenging and difficult. These challenges, if dealt with appropriately, can also be some of the most rewarding experiences for the nurse and indeed patients/service users. There is a requirement for nurses, in particular, to be self-aware and monitor their reactions in these situations, remembering that they are involved in professional relationships and not personal ones. Some behaviours are not acceptable or tolerated, and their consequences would be seen as professional misconduct.

CHAPTER 1

Professional skills and accountability

Tina Moore

Overview

The 'duty of candour' is a professional and statutory requirement (Care Quality Commission [CQC]) that every healthcare professional must be open and honest with patients when something that goes wrong with their treatment or care causes, or has the potential to cause, harm or distress. They must refrain from preventing the escalation of concerns and encourage a learning culture by reporting errors.

The Nursing and Midwifery Council (2019b) state that healthcare professionals must:

- tell the patient (or, where appropriate, the patient's advocate, carer or family) when something has gone wrong
- apologise to the patient (or, where appropriate, the patient's advocate, carer or family)
- offer an appropriate remedy or support to put matters right (if possible)
- explain fully to the patient (or, where appropriate, the patient's advocate, carer or family) the short- and long-term effects of what has happened. (NMC, 2019b)

Link to *Future Nurse Proficiencies* (NMC 2018a)

Platform 1 Being an accountable profession: specifically 1.1, 1.5, 1.9, 1.17.

Expected knowledge

- Understanding of *The Code: Professional Standards of Practice and Behaviour for Nurses, Midwives and Nursing Associates* (NMC 2018b)
- Knowing the role of a student nurse
- An overview of a qualified nurse on the professional register

Introduction

Nursing practice demands that all nurses are competent and strive towards developing mastery in their chosen fields. This principle should also hold a genuine passion and vision for nursing, coupled with an endeavour towards excellence and quality. If a nurse fails to follow 'The Code' (NMC 2018b), they may be reported to the NMC for an investigation into their 'fitness to practise'.

Accountability is an integral part of professional practice, requiring the nurse to explain and justify their actions and omissions in relation to care. Definitions of accountability reflect the expectation that justification should be evidence based.

Content

Professional skills	Accountability	Delegation
Managing the clinical environment	Record keeping	Revalidation

Learning outcomes

- Understand the term 'duty of candour' and its implications for nurses
- Identify relevant professional standards
- Discuss the meaning of accountability and how this relates to the nurse
- Consider the principles of delegation
- Give a rationale and outline the processes in managing a ward or environment that delivers patient care

Key background

Today, we are experiencing the changes in role boundaries between nurses and other professional groups, particularly those in the medical field. In response the profession must continually be professionally accountable for expanding their clinical skill set and consistently implementing a high-quality evidence-based approach to clinical practice. Ongoing clinical competency development requires active participation to attain, maintain and develop further the skills necessary to provide outstanding care for the patient/service user population. This is to encourage patients to have confidence in the ability of nurses. Through this it is anticipated that occurrences that test our duty of candour will be reduced.

Over recent years the profession has seen a reduction in qualified staff and an increase in nursing associate roles/healthcare support workers. Nursing associates and healthcare support workers are undertaking many of the tasks usually done by registered nurses. Even between 'nurses', the boundaries of their roles have become unclear. This situation has also seen an increase in delegated duties from qualified nurses to those not or less qualified, including student nurses. This has presented further concerns and confusion for nurses around accountability issues relating to delegation.

Nurses, as healthcare professionals and the organisations to which they belong, are accountable to civil and criminal courts to ensure that their services and performances meet legal requirements. They are also, as employees, accountable to their employer under their contract of duty. In addition, nurses are accountable to their professional body, the Nursing and Midwifery Council, in maintaining the patient's safety.

There is a legal and professional duty of care owed to patients by nurses at all levels. This is part of the tort of negligence that is designed to protect the patient's safety. The key factor is the standard of care expected of practitioners (including nurses) performing particular roles and the competency of the practitioner to perform to that standard. Practitioners must inform a senior staff member if they are unable to perform competently.

PROFESSIONAL SKILLS

To be a professional is to be engaged in activities that are guided by a body of knowledge and evidence.

Compassion in Practice (Department of Health 2012) identifies 6 core values (known as the 6 Cs) Care, Compassion, Competence, Communication, Courage and Commitment.

The underpinning principles are:
> Helping people to stay independent, maximising well-being and improving health outcomes.
> Working with people to provide a positive experience of care.
> Delivering high-quality care and measuring the impact of care.
> Building and strengthening leadership.
> Ensuring that there is the right staff with the right skills in the right place.
> Supporting positive staff experiences.

Principles of nursing practice

All nurses should:

A. Treat everyone with dignity and humanity. Understand their individual needs, show compassion and sensitivity, and provide care in a respectful and equal way.
B. Take responsibility for the care they provide and answer for their own judgments and actions. Care should be carried out in agreement with the patients, their families and carers and should also meet professional body and the legal requirements.
C. Manage risks, be vigilant about risk, and help to keep everyone safe in the places they receive health care.
D. Provide and promote care putting people at the centre, involving patients and their significant others in decisions, helping them make informed choices about treatment and care.
E. Be at the centre communication process: assessing, recording and reporting on treatment and care, handling information sensitively and confidentially, dealing with complaints effectively, and conscientiously report issues they are concerned about.
F. Have up-to-date knowledge and skills, and use these with intelligence, insight and understanding in line with the needs of each individual in their care.
G. Work closely with their own team and with other professionals, making sure patients' care and treatment is co-ordinated, is of a high standard and has the best possible outcome.
H. Lead by example, develop themselves and other staff, and influence the way care is given in a manner that is open and responds to individual needs.

(Adapted from RCN 2010)

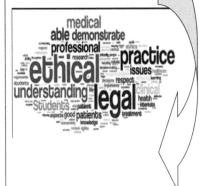

Ethical considerations in practice
The Royal College of Nursing have produced a toolkit to facilitate and support ethical considerations within nursing practice. It is specifically designed to support ethical decision making for patients who are dying. However, the principles can be transferred to any clinical situation.
The 5 themes are:
1. Establish the relevant clinical facts of the case.
2. Assess the wishes of the patient and those important to them.
3. Consider the legal perspectives.
4. Consider the ethical perspectives.
5. Be aware of the processes needed to support the decision making.

FIGURE 1.1 Professional skills

ACCOUNTABILITY

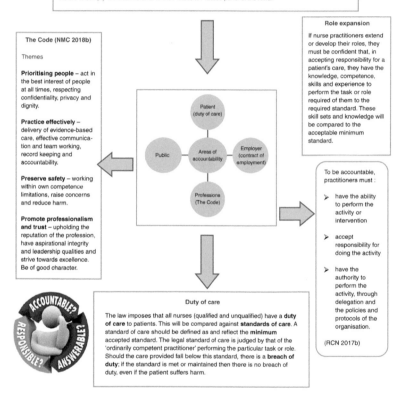

Professional accountability

Nurses must be professionally accountable for expanding their clinical skill set and consistently implement high-standard, evidence-based practice findings to guide nursing interventions. Ongoing clinical competency requires active participation to attain and maintain the skills necessary to provide exceptional care for patients.

Professional accountability underpins safe practice and requires the nurse to take ownership of and provide justification in relation to patient care and clinical decision making.

Failure to comply will mean referral to the Fitness to Practice panel of the NMC.

The Code (NMC 2018b)

Themes

Prioritising people – act in the best interest of people at all times, respecting confidentiality, privacy and dignity.

Practice effectively – delivery of evidence-based care, effective communication and team working, record keeping and accountability.

Preserve safety – working within own competence limitations, raise concerns and reduce harm.

Promote professionalism and trust – upholding the reputation of the profession, have aspirational integrity and leadership qualities and strive towards excellence. Be of good character.

Role expansion

If nurse practitioners extend or develop their roles, they must be confident that, in accepting responsibility for a patient's care, they have the knowledge, competence, skills and experience to perform the task or role required of them to the required standard. These skill sets and knowledge will be compared to the acceptable minimum standard.

To be accountable, practitioners must :

➢ have the ability to perform the activity or intervention

➢ accept responsibility for doing the activity

➢ have the authority to perform the activity, through delegation and the policies and protocols of the organisation.

(RCN 2017b)

Patient (duty of care)

Public

Areas of accountability

Employer (contract of employment)

Professions (The Code)

Duty of care

The law imposes that all nurses (qualified and unqualified) have a **duty of care** to patients. This will be compared against **standards of care**. A standard of care should be defined as and reflect the **minimum** accepted standard. The legal standard of care is judged by that of the 'ordinarily competent practitioner' performing the particular task or role. Should the care provided fall below this standard, there is a **breach of duty**; if the standard is met or maintained then there is no breach of duty, even if the patient suffers harm.

ACCOUNTABLE? RESPONSIBLE? ANSWERABLE?

FIGURE 1.2 Accountability

DELEGATION

Delegation

With delegation, there is a transfer of tasks to be performed by another individual (the delegatee). This individual accepts responsibility for carrying out the delegated work and is accountable as to how the work is carried out. The accountability and responsibility still remain with the delegator who needs to be sure that the work is delegated appropriately. The delegator is also accountable for their decision making in relation to the delegation.

Five 'rights' of delegation

➢ Right task
➢ Right circumstances
➢ Right person
➢ Right supervision
➢ Right direction and communication

(National Council of State Boards 1995)

Ensure that:

❖ delegation does not harm the interests of people in your care
❖ the task is within the other person's scope of competence
❖ the person you are delegating to understands the boundaries of their own competence
❖ the person you are delegating to understands the task
❖ the person you are delegating to understands clearly the circumstances in which they must refer back to you
❖ you take reasonable steps to identify any risks and whether any supervision might be necessary
❖ reasonable steps are taken to monitor the outcome of the delegated task.

(NMC 2018c)

As a delegator you should:

➢ only delegate tasks and duties that are within the other person's scope of competence, making sure that they fully understand the instructions

➢ make sure that everyone you delegate tasks to is adequately supervised and supported so they can provide safe and compassionate care

➢ check and confirm that the outcome of any task delegated to someone else meets the required standard

(NMC 2018c)

Accepting delegated tasks

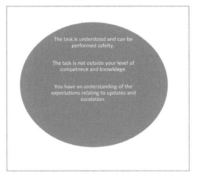

The task is understood and can be performed safelty.

The task is not outside your level of competnece and knowledge.

You have an understanding of the expectations relating to updates and escalation.

Key principles of delegation

- Delegation decisions should be made in the best interest of the patient.
- Individuals accepting delegation should be suitably trained to undertake the task.
- Evidence of the delegatee's competence should be assessed and documented.
- The role/delegated tasks should be within the delegatee's role description.
- Clear protocols and policies in place to guide clinical judgement and decision making.
- The team should be made aware that the task has been delegated.
- There must be appropriate levels of supervision by the person who has delegated the task and feedback provided.
- The whole process should be assessed and monitored in order to identify risks.

FIGURE 1.3 Delegation

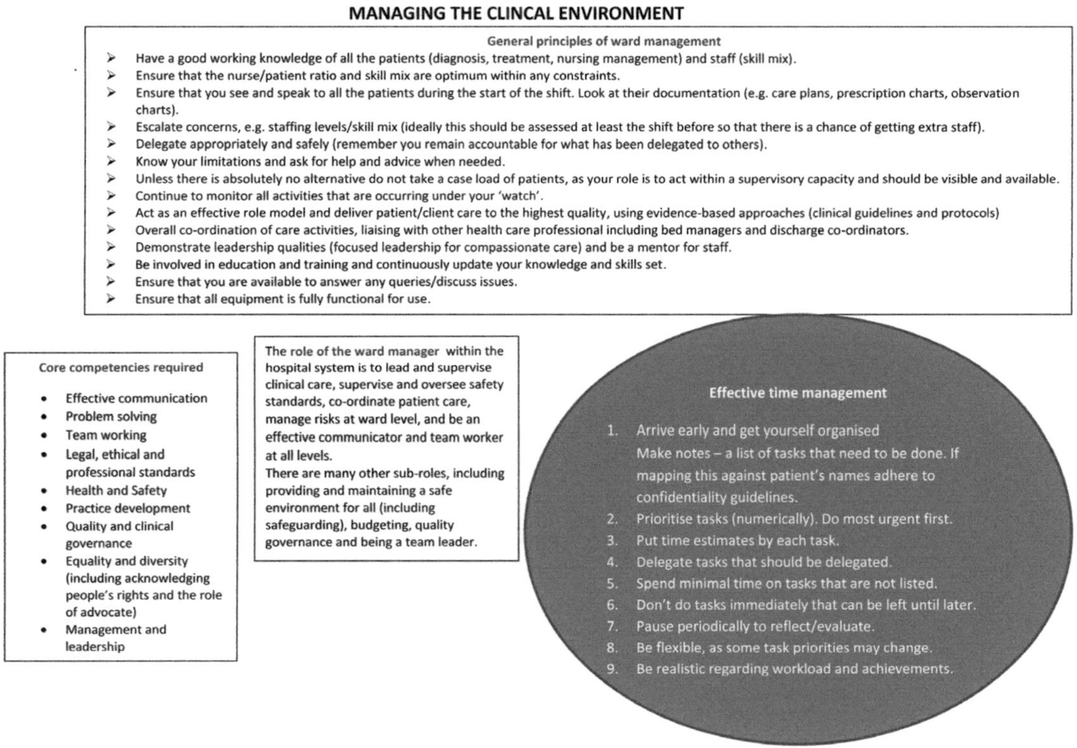

MANAGING THE CLINICAL ENVIRONMENT

General principles of ward management

➤ Have a good working knowledge of all the patients (diagnosis, treatment, nursing management) and staff (skill mix).
➤ Ensure that the nurse/patient ratio and skill mix are optimum within any constraints.
➤ Ensure that you see and speak to all the patients during the start of the shift. Look at their documentation (e.g. care plans, prescription charts, observation charts).
➤ Escalate concerns, e.g. staffing levels/skill mix (ideally this should be assessed at least the shift before so that there is a chance of getting extra staff).
➤ Delegate appropriately and safely (remember you remain accountable for what has been delegated to others).
➤ Know your limitations and ask for help and advice when needed.
➤ Unless there is absolutely no alternative do not take a case load of patients, as your role is to act within a supervisory capacity and should be visible and available.
➤ Continue to monitor all activities that are occurring under your 'watch'.
➤ Act as an effective role model and deliver patient/client care to the highest quality, using evidence-based approaches (clinical guidelines and protocols).
➤ Overall co-ordination of care activities, liaising with other health care professional including bed managers and discharge co-ordinators.
➤ Demonstrate leadership qualities (focused leadership for compassionate care) and be a mentor for staff.
➤ Be involved in education and training and continuously update your knowledge and skills set.
➤ Ensure that you are available to answer any queries/discuss issues.
➤ Ensure that all equipment is fully functional for use.

Effective time management

1. Arrive early and get yourself organised
   Make notes – a list of tasks that need to be done. If mapping this against patient's names adhere to confidentiality guidelines.
2. Prioritise tasks (numerically). Do most urgent first.
   Put time estimates by each task.
3. Delegate tasks that should be delegated.
4. Delegate tasks that can be left until later.
5. Spend minimal time on tasks that are not listed.
6. Don't do tasks immediately that can be left until later.
7. Pause periodically to reflect/evaluate.
8. Be flexible, as some task priorities may change.
9. Be realistic regarding workload and achievements.

Core competencies required

- Effective communication
- Problem solving
- Team working
- Legal, ethical and professional standards
- Health and Safety
- Practice development
- Quality and clinical governance
- Equality and diversity (including acknowledging people's rights and the role of advocate)
- Management and leadership

The role of the ward manager within the hospital system is to lead and supervise clinical care, supervise and oversee safety standards, co-ordinate patient care, manage risks at ward level, and be an effective communicator and team worker at all levels.
There are many other sub-roles, including providing and maintaining a safe environment for all (including safeguarding), budgeting, quality governance and being a team leader.

FIGURE 1.4 Managing the clinical environment

RECORD KEEPING

Record keeping

Record keeping is the organisation and storage of all documents, either hand-written or digital, in relation to patient/service user care. Its key purpose is to produce an account of that care and treatment as part of the nurse's duty of care.

Wherever possible records should be written with the involvement of the patient/service user and or carer.

Challenges

➤ Nurses are subject to increasing scrutiny of their record keeping

➤ Nurses registrations are being discontinued because of poor record keeping

➤ Patients are increasingly more willing to complain about their care

➤ Amid the stress of a busy day, record keeping may not be completed, or not be completed as well or thoroughly as it should be

➤ If record keeping is seen as a 'chore' then there is a risk of standards being compromised

➤ Poor record keeping may indicate:
  - Poor professional standards
  - Inadequate assessment
  - Inadequate care management
  - Inadequate communication.

Professional expectations

- Keep clear, accurate and relevant records that are based on facts, not assumptions or opinions
- Complete all records in a timely manner
- Make sure all records are clear and professionally written
- Do not use unnecessary abbreviations
- Identify risks/problems and what has been done to deal with them
- Do not falsify records, take immediate and appropriate action if you become aware that someone has not kept to this requirement
- Ensure records are clearly written, dated, timed and signed
- Do not erase or delete entries – just put a single line through the information and record as an error
- Records should be readable when photocopied or scanned
- Provide clear evidence of care that is planned/delivered – share decision making
- Ensure that all records are kept securely
- Collect, treat and store all date appropriately

Quality records will:

Make clear decision-making processes in patient care management

Support effective clinical decision making and judgements, and ensure continuity of care

Facilitate communication between health care professionals

Identify risks and early detection of problems

Help in the complaints procedure

Support clinical audit, research, allocation of resources and performance planning

Legal obligations of record keeping

1. *The Public Records Act (1958)* – Sets out broad responsibilities for NHS staff

2. *The Data Protection Act (1998)* – regulates the management of personal information held

3. *The Freedom of Information Act (2000)* – right of access to recorded information

4. The Common Law Duty of Confidentiality – legal duty, not documented in any single publication

5. *The NHS Confidentiality Code of Practice* – guidance

6. *Manual for Caldicott Guardians* (Bunch 2017) – provides guidance to the organisation's senior person overseeing the appropriate, legal and ethical use of information

FIGURE 1.5 Record keeping

REVALIDATION

Revalidation is the process towards a nurse maintaining and renewing their entry on the professional register. Renewal is every three years. The purpose of revalidation is to improve and preserve public protection by making sure that nurses remain 'fit to practise' throughout their career. So, revalidation:

- reinforces the nurse's duty to maintain their fitness to practise within their own scope of practice and helps maintain safe and effective practice
- encourages the incorporation of the Code in everyday practices, professional and personal development
- encourages engagement in professional networks and discussions and can help to reduce professional isolation
- enhances employer engagement in NMC regulatory standards and increases access and participation in appraisals and continuing professional development.

(RCN 2019)

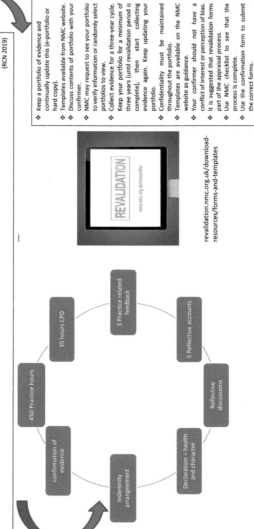

revalidation.nmc.org.uk/download-resources/forms-and-templates

- ❖ Keep a portfolio of evidence and continually update this (e-portfolio or hard copy).
- ❖ Templates available from NMC website.
- ❖ Discuss contents of portfolio with your confirmer.
- ❖ NMC may request to see your portfolio to verify information or randomly select portfolios to view.
- ❖ Collect evidence for a three-year cycle. Keep your portfolio for a minimum of three years (until revalidation period is complete), then start collecting evidence again. Keep updating your portfolio.
- ❖ Confidentiality must be maintained throughout the portfolio.
- ❖ Templates are available on the NMC website as guidance.
- ❖ Your confirmer should not have a conflict of interest or perception of bias.
- ❖ It is suggested that revalidation forms part of the appraisal process.
- ❖ Use NMC checklist to see that the process is complete.
- ❖ Use the confirmation form to submit the correct forms.

(NMC 2019a)

FIGURE 1.6 Revalidation

Activity: now test yourself

1 List the five rights of delegation

2 State whether true or false

    a The main reason for delegating tasks is when you have no time to complete them

    b Accountability cannot be delegated

    c There should be clear protocols in place to help guide accountability

3 What are the three criteria for nurses to be accountable

4 What are the competencies of an effective ward manager?:

    a Effective communication, problem solving, quality and clinical governance

    b Problem solving, quality and clinical governance, equality and diversity

    c Quality and clinical governance, equality and diversity, leadership

    d Management and leadership, problem solving, budgeting

5 Write down what criteria you would use as examples of good documentation/record keeping if you were to undertake an audit

Answers

1   Five rights of delegation are:

Right task
Right circumstances
Right person
Right supervision
Right direction and communication

2   a   False
Delegation should be done in the best interest of the patient. The delegatee should have the appropriate skills and knowledge to undertake the task successfully. They should fully understand the instructions.

b   True
Accountability cannot be delegated.

c   True
There should be clear protocols in place to help guide accountability.

3   To be accountable nurses must:

have the ability to perform the activity or intervention
accept responsibility for doing the activity
have the authority to perform the activity, through delegation and the policies and protocols of the organisation

4   All competencies are required – a, b, c, d

5   Any of the following:

- *clear, accurate, professionally written and relevant records that are based on facts*
- *completed in timely manner*
- *no unnecessary abbreviations*
- *no spelling or grammatical errors*
- *written in English*
- *risks/problems clearly identified and what actions taken*
- *legal requirements upheld*
- *writing is legible and entries are dated, timed and signed*

- *for errors – a single line through the information and recorded as an error*
- evidence of care that is planned/delivered; decision-making is transparent
- records are kept securely

Reflection: ask yourself

1   What do I know that I did not know before?

2   What I am confused about now?

3   What areas do I need to focus on?

4   My action plan for further learning (make objectives SMART: specific, measurable, achievable, realist and timeframe)

CHAPTER 2

Communication

Sheila Cunningham

Overview

The NMC (2018a) indicate that nurses must be aware of and practise evidence-based, best practice approaches to communication for supporting people of all ages, and their families and carers, in preventing ill health and managing their care. Furthermore these skills extend to working with people in professional teams.

Expected knowledge

- Episodes or encounters where communication is required
- Physiology of hearing, speaking and information processing

Link to *Future Nurse Proficiencies* (NMC 2018a)

Throughout all Platforms 1–7
Annexe A: communication and relationship management skills (all points from 1 to 4). Effective communication is central to the provision of safe and compassionate person-centred care. Registered nurses in all fields of nursing practice must be able to demonstrate the ability to communicate and manage relationships with people of all ages with a range of mental, physical, cognitive and behavioural health challenges.

Introduction

Communication is a reciprocal process that involves the exchange of verbal and non-verbal messages to convey feelings, information, ideas and knowledge. As nurses we have a responsibility to include good communication and psychological support, developing skills to enable this, which is as important as developing technological skills. It is core to nursing care and supporting humans within our care.

Content

The humanistic approach to communication	Skills for effective communication	Empathy and addressing sensory challenges
Professional communication	Active listening	Context of communication

Learning outcomes

- Describe and apply humanistic approach to communication in practice
- Decide how to enhance communication across the lifespan by using the appropriate skills
- Understand the importance of empathy when caring for patients across the fields, and for their families and carers
- Identify and suggest means to promote communication in people with challenging or impaired conditions
- Reflect on your own communication skills and ways to enhance them

Key background

Nursing involves working with a wide range of people across the lifespan, within a multicultural society, often when they are at their most vulnerable. Feeling vulnerable can lead people to behave in ways that may be challenging and difficult.

Communication underpins skills for assessing, planning, providing and managing evidence-based, best practice, nursing care. This is because a diverse range of communication and relationship management skills is required to ensure that individuals, their families and their carers are actively involved in and understand care decisions. These skills are vital when making accurate, culturally aware assessments of care needs and ensuring that the needs, priorities, expertise and preferences of people are always valued and taken into account.

As professionals we have a duty to make care person centred, and this includes communication. When people have special communication needs or a disability, it is essential that reasonable adjustments be made to communicate, provide and share information in a manner that promotes optimum understanding and engagement, and facilitates equal access to high-quality care (NMC 2018b). Communication is more than imparting messages; it is also making connections. Communication failure, such as failing to introduce oneself, can occur when staff regard patients as a series of symptoms and tasks, or time pressures and thoughtless rushed encounters of garbled messages. Treating people as humans with social and emotional needs is paramount to all communication skills as well as not unintentionally leaving patients feeling dehumanised. This is not in the spirit of person-centred care and can be addressed with simple measures (such as introducing yourself) with huge beneficial effects.

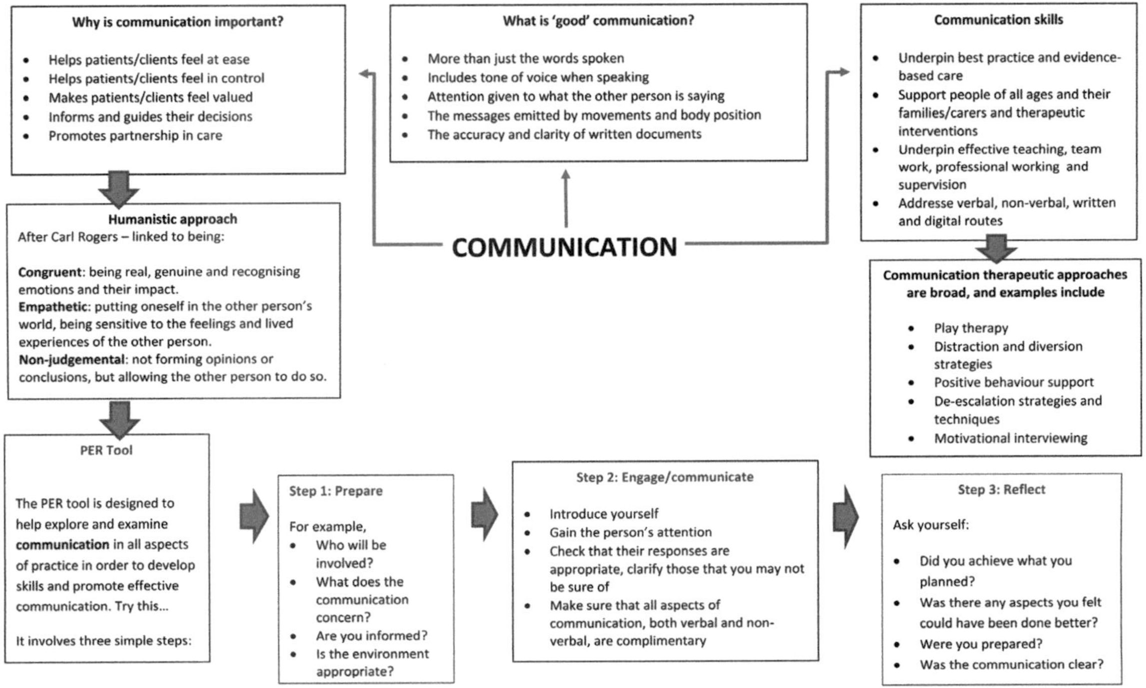

COMMUNICATION

What is 'good' communication?

- More than just the words spoken
- Includes tone of voice when speaking
- Attention given to what the other person is saying
- The messages emitted by movements and body position
- The accuracy and clarity of written documents

Why is communication important?

- Helps patients/clients feel at ease
- Helps patients/clients feel in control
- Makes patients/clients feel valued
- Informs and guides their decisions
- Promotes partnership in care

Humanistic approach

After Carl Rogers – linked to being:

Congruent: being real, genuine and recognising emotions and their impact.

Empathetic: putting oneself in the other person's world, being sensitive to the feelings and lived experiences of the other person.

Non-judgemental: not forming opinions or conclusions, but allowing the other person to do so.

PER Tool

The PER tool is designed to help explore and examine communication in all aspects of practice in order to develop skills and promote effective communication. Try this...

It involves three simple steps:

Step 1: Prepare

For example,

- Who will be involved?
- What does the communication concern?
- Are you informed?
- Is the environment appropriate?

Step 2: Engage/communicate

- Introduce yourself
- Gain the person's attention
- Check that their responses are appropriate, clarify those that you may not be sure of
- Make sure that all aspects of communication, both verbal and non-verbal, are complimentary

Step 3: Reflect

Ask yourself:

- Did you achieve what you planned?
- Were there any aspects you felt could have been done better?
- Were you prepared?
- Was the communication clear?

Communication skills

- Underpin best practice and evidence-based care
- Support people of all ages and their families/carers and therapeutic interventions
- Underpin effective teaching, team work, professional working and supervision
- Address verbal, non-verbal, written and digital routes

Communication therapeutic approaches are broad, and examples include

- Play therapy
- Distraction and diversion strategies
- Positive behaviour support
- De-escalation strategies and techniques
- Motivational interviewing

FIGURE 2.1 Communication overview

USING COMMUNICATION IN PRACTICE

Communicating with professionals

Mentors/supervisors
- Expressing interest, motivation and being professional through asking questions, being proactive, being safe and tailoring communication to the recipient.

Wider team
- Awareness of each professional's role, what needs to be communicated and when, ensuring clarity in communicating about patients by using techniques such as SBAR:
Situation – what the communication concerns
Background – essential details
Assessment – of the issue
Recommendation – how it ought to be addressed.

Telephone communication

Requires the same skills but requires judgement due to:
1. lack of visual cues in communicating
2. purpose of the telephone interaction
3. vigilance for safety and confidentiality.

Telephone communication with professionals
- Establish identity (you and them).
- Be clear (use SBAR if necessary).
- Document if necessary.

Messages
Be aware of confidentiality and storing messages.

Nursing triage
This requires advanced skills and further training of telephone communication.

Record keeping and communication

- Vital part of effective communication in nursing.
- Integral to promoting safety and continuity of care.

Key principles for documents
- Completed as soon as possible
- Signed, timed and dated (handwritten), or traceable to the person completing it (digital)
- Completed accurately
- Free from jargon or speculation
- In clear, plain English
- Legible
- IF alterations needed, the original entry must remain visible (draw a single line through the record) and the new entry must be signed, timed and dated
- Stored securely and for as long as local policy stipulates (requires knowledge of legislation and of digital storage systems)

Social media

The Code (NMC 2018b) states:
'Use all forms of spoken, written and digital communication (including social media and networking sites) responsibly' (para 20.10). The guidance is to:
- be informed
- think before you post
- protect your professionalism and your reputation.

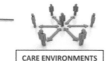

CARE ENVIRONMENTS

Adult nursing

People aged 18 years upwards.
- Ask patient what they wish to be called.
- Assess their communication and how their care/treatment will affect this (i.e. if unconscious, need communication aids, language restrictions).
- Be aware of where conversations occur (with or about patients/clients).
- Communication is partnership and requires trust and openness.

Child and young person nursing

communication varies depending on development stages.
- For younger children, appropriate touch and facial expressions are important in non-verbal communication for trust and caring expression.
- Impaired abilities may impact on usual developmental stages so communication is also individual.

Mental health nursing

Advanced skills for therapeutic approaches.
- Depending on their problem, clients may need clarifying thoughts and communication.
- Vulnerability of these patients/clients is related to their ability to communicate or understand communications due to their mental health state.
- Attention to signs expressed in verbal and non-verbal behaviour is core to care.

FIGURE 2.2 Communication in practice

COMMUNICATION SKILLS: DETAILS

Verbal skills

Language: vocabulary choice. Miscommunication may arise due to:
- 'bad language' or swearing (reflect on whether this is the words or the emotions being communicated?)
- expressions being perceived as belonging to a particular social group
- words not being used in communication (e.g. young people and sensitive topics)
- use of complex terminology (medical/therapy terms).

Paralanguage: the way words are said, which impacts interpretation.
- Includes pitch, volume, rate, tone and intonation. Also considers dialect and accent.

Non-verbal skills

Potentially the most influential aspect, and often people lack self-awareness of their non-verbal skills.
- **Head movements** can reinforce or strengthen verbal communication or agreement.
- **Facial expressions** may express additional aspects such as emotions or empathy.
- **Eye contact** is important to express emotion and concern, but may be misinterpreted in varying cultures, requiring awareness of this.
- **Proximity and orientation**, referring to body position, distance, and contact, may express interest or disinterest, power, or defensiveness/aggression. Sensitivity is required to address the right message.
- **Touch**, whilst essential in nursing, is subject to different social and cultural rules about permissions or what is appropriate for age, culture or genders of clients.

Aspects of communication skills

The Humanistic philosophical approach outlined earlier underpins practical and cultural aspects of communication. These guide interactions to communicate effectively.

Communication can be said to fall into four categories:

1. Verbal skills (language and paralanguage)
2. Non-verbal skills
3. Perceptions and judgements
4. Alternative techniques for sensory impairment

Tips... verbal communication

- Keep verbal communication simple and to the point.
- Ensure client/patient is listening.
- Use terms the patient/client understands.
- Check understanding with open questions.
- Be aware of unconscious bias.

Active listening

- Challenging in busy clinical areas.

Consider:
- Stay focused and attentive
- Face the person, look interested
- Detect emotions
- Ask questions to clarify
- Don't interrupt
- Embrace silence if needed
- Summarise key facts
- Be non judgmental

Perceptions and judgements
(by patients/clients, by other professionals, by colleagues)

These are formed from:
- observation of nurses during their work
- nurses' verbal and non-verbal skills
- personal characteristics
- appearance, professional dress and behaviour

This necessitates awareness of these aspects and their implications for effective communication.

The SOLER position

Egan (2010, p.135) identifies certain non-verbal skills summarised in the acronym **SOLER**:

Sitting facing the client squarely, at an angle.
Adopting an Open posture, arms and legs uncrossed.
Leaning (at times) towards the person.
Maintaining good Eye contact, without staring.
Relaxed posture.

FIGURE 2.3 Communication: verbal and non-verbal

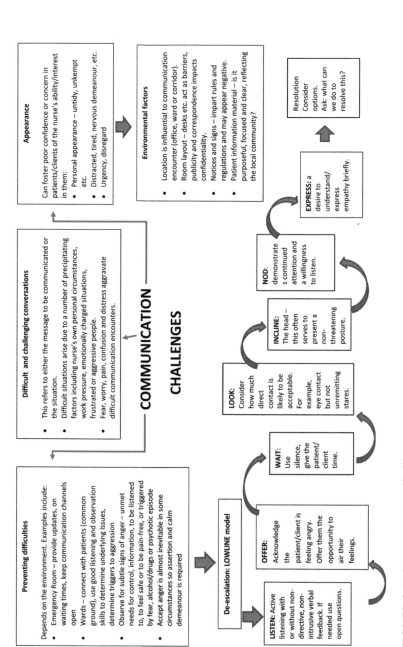

Appearance

Can foster poor confidence or concern in patients/clients of the nurse's ability/interest in them:

- Personal appearance – untidy, unkempt etc.
- Distracted, tired, nervous demeanour, etc.
- Urgency, disregard

Difficult and challenging conversations

- This refers to either the message to be communicated or the situation.
- Difficult situations arise due to a number of precipitating factors including nurse's own personal circumstances, work pressure, emotionally charged situations, frustrated or aggressive people.
- Fear, worry, pain, confusion and distress aggravate difficult communication encounters.

Environmental factors

- Location is influential to communication encounter (office, ward or corridor).
- Room layout – desks etc. act as barriers, publicity and correspondence impacts confidentiality.
- Notices and signs – impart rules and regulations and may appear negative.
- Patient information material – is it purposeful, focused and clear, reflecting the local community?

COMMUNICATION

CHALLENGES

Preventing difficulties

Depends on the environment. Examples include:

- Emergency Room – provide updates, on waiting times, keep communication channels open
- Wards – connect with patients (common ground), use good listening and observation skills to determine underlying issues, determine triggers to aggression
- Observe for subtle signs of anger – unmet needs for control, information, to be listened to, to feel safe or to be pain-free, or triggered by fear, alcohol/drugs or psychotic episode
- Accept anger is almost inevitable in some circumstances so assertion and calm demeanour is required

De-escalation: LOWLINE model

LISTEN: Active listening with or without non-directive, non-intrusive verbal feedback. If needed use open questions.

OFFER: Acknowledge the patient/client is feeling angry. Offer them the opportunity to air their feelings.

WAIT: Use silence, give the patient/client time.

LOOK: Consider how much direct contact is likely to be acceptable. For example, eye contact but not unremitting stares.

INCLINE: The head – this often serves to present a non-threatening posture.

NOD: demonstrates continued attention and a willingness to listen.

EXPRESS: a desire to understand/express empathy briefly.

Resolution Consider options. Ask: what can we do to resolve this?

FIGURE 2.4 Communication challenges

Sensory impairment extent

Varies from mild to severe
May be progressive (elderly) or from an early age
Can be isolating so careful attention to communication is essential
Aids adopted include (examples, not exhaustive):
- hearing aids
- lip reading
- relying on other senses (e.g. if blind then listening more acutely)
- glasses
- alterative provision (e.g. Braille, font size, coloured background to resources).

Sensory impairments and communication

- Everyone communicates differently, and for professionals (or anyone) communication skills continually develop.
- Multi-sensory impairment (or MSI) refers to a person (child or adult) who has impairments with both sight and hearing. Children with MSI may also have cognitive, medical or physical disabilities, and challenges which affect the other senses (Murdoch 2009).
- For people with MSI, specific methods of communication may be required.
- If impairment is serious, specialist training and experience may be needed.

COMMUNICATION: SENSORY ISSUES

Communication preparation suggestions

- Make sure you have the person's attention before trying to communicate with them, e.g. gently touching their arm, if appropriate, or saying their name.
- Identify yourself clearly. For some individuals, spelling out your name using the deafblind manual may also be appropriate. Check that you are in the best position to communicate.
- Try to make a connection. If eye contact is difficult offer your hands for the person to touch.
- Be aware of the environment and adapt the conditions to suit the individual you are communicating with, e.g. noise, light, space.
- When using 'signing', consider your clothing – high-contrast colours to your skin tone may be helpful, but confusing patterns (e.g. zigzags) can make it more difficult for the person to define your signs.
- Speak clearly and a little slower without shouting.
- Use clear lip patterns and enunciation but without over-exaggerating.
- Keep your face visible, e.g. avoid smoking, eating or wearing masks.
- Use gestures and facial expressions to support what you are saying.
- Repeat phrases or re-phrase sentences, if necessary.
- Try writing things down or using pictures, photos, drawings or objects as props to help explain or reinforce what you are saying. Tablets or phones are another good way of offering images to support communication.
- For phone conversations, consider using a text relay service such as Next Generation Text (https://www.ngts.org.uk/).

Persons with dementia: tips and aspects of conversations to avoid

1. *Remember when ... ?* This can be a frustrating or painful experience, best to lead the conversation and allow the person to join in. What about saying 'I remember when¼' instead? That way the person can search their memory calmly without feeling embarrassed, then join in if they like.

2. *I've just told you that* This phrase only reminds the person of their condition. Try to be polite and as patient as possible.

3. *Your brother died 10 years ago*' Reminding them of a loved one's death can be painful, even causing them to relive the grief they've already experienced. Try showing sensitivity. Seek advice from specialists.

4. *What did you do this morning?*' Too many open-ended questions can be stressful. Encourage choices but with more focused questions, e.g. instead of 'do you want tea or coffee?', more simply ask 'do you want a cup of tea?'

5. *Let's have a cup of tea now, then after that we can go for nice in the park you like.*' This is too open and complex, better to give directions or instructions one step at a time.

6. *Do you need some help with that, love?*' Words like these, 'love' etc., can be patronising for people living with dementia, and this causes older people to feel infantilised. Instead ensure their dignity and respect is maintained, and use their name (recognising the person).

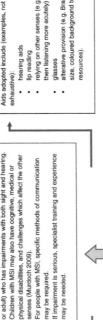

FIGURE 2.5 Additional communication skills

Activity: now test yourself

1   Why is communication important?

2   What steps are there in the PER tool of communication and how can one apply them?

3   Identify one communication challenge that a nurse or healthcare professional might encounter in practice and how this can be addressed

4   Which of the following does non-verbal communication NOT include?:

   a   facial expressions

   b   eye contact

   c   physical touch

   d   body position

   e   none of the above

5   Asking open questions is important in communication. Why might this pose a challenge to someone with dementia?

6   What is meant by 'multisensory impairment' and how might this impact on effective communication?

Answers

1   To support people in our care, to empower and enable them, to make decisions, to convey feelings, needs, emotions, etc.

2   P: prepare
     E: engage
     R: reflect
     These steps can be used in every encounter with a person in our care – to ensure that communication is effective and planned to be useful, for example when engaging with tasks or skills such as advising new parents on breastfeeding or weaning, or supporting and preparing someone to go home after a hospital stay – any and all encounters that are within our caring remit.

3   There are a huge number to choose form, such as difficult conversations about death, bereavement or bad news; dealing with people in pain or who are confused, angry people who feel unheard or even colleagues in emotionally charged situations.
     The key to address these is to recognise that there may be underpinning issues – unmet needs, frustrations, etc. – and acknowledge them. Seek a resolution in a positive way and if needed use a de-escalation approach to enable this.

4   e   none of the above
     They are all non-verbal elements reminding us that body movements, expressions and gestures all add to communication transmission as well as interpretation of messages.

5   This may cause confusion and frustration if the ability to select options or cognitive processes is slow. It is best to assess the person's capacity to process the information and be patient with meeting needs, and have simple straightforward communication, perhaps offering choices requiring yes or no responses if severe challenges are evident.

6   This refers to hearing, visual or cognitive impairments that impact on the diverse elements of communication. This may result in adopting supplementary strategies to aid

communication – writing down points or messages, using lip-reading approaches, hearing aids or even technology such as voice-to-text services, whatever is appropriate, age and impairment specific, and available. Seeking specialist guidance and help are also a sensible option.

Reflection: ask yourself

1   What do I know now that I didn't know before?

2   What am I confused/unclear about?

3   What areas do I need to focus on?

4   My action plan for further learning (make objectives SMART)

CHAPTER 3

The nursing process

Tina Moore

Overview

In general, the overall goals of nursing are to: promote, maintain or restore health or, in the case of terminal illness, to achieve a peaceful death; enable people to manage their own health care; provide cost-effective, quality care; continue to find ways of improving satisfaction with health-care delivery. Frameworks used within nursing go some way to providing direction for the achievement of these goals.

Link to *Future Nurse Proficiencies* (NMC 2018a)

Platform 3 Assessing needs and planning care: specifically 3.4, 3.5, 3.15
Platform 7 Co-ordinating care: specifically 7.10

Expected knowledge

- An overview of the use of frameworks to guide nursing practice
- Some models for nursing, e.g. model of Roper, Logan and Tierney, Casey model, and Peplau model

Introduction

Frameworks have been used within nursing for a long time. Their main function are to provide some structure to the assessment and provision of care. One example of such a framework is the nursing model. There are a number of nursing models in existence (mostly from North America) that outline the author's view of what nursing should be. Many of these nursing models are the result of fairly extensive research. So, a lot of thought and evidence gathering have been used in their creation. It is outside the remit of this particular book to discuss these models in detail. But the point being made here is that the nursing model should be used together with the nursing process. The nursing process is a systematic, problem-solving approach that provides structure for the implementation of a nursing model. The use of frameworks is necessary to gather relevant, appropriate and thorough patient information and help with clinical reasoning, clinical judgement and decision-making.

Content

Admission, transfer, discharge	Nursing process	Assessment
Planning	Implementation	Evaluation

Learning outcomes

- Outline and differentiate the stages of the nursing process
- Explore and examine each stage individually and how this relates to patient care
- Utilise the nursing process to provide a framework of care within clinical practice
- Discuss the role of the nurse in relation to the process of admission and discharge

Key background

The nursing process is an organised, systematic approach to the management of patient care. It consists of five sequential and interrelated stages. These stages are: assessment, diagnosis, planning, implementation and evaluation. These stages of the nursing process are viewed as holistic but interconnected with each other to create a whole.

Nursing diagnosis is a relatively recent addition in the UK and complements the efforts towards making nursing a respectful and professional discipline. In addition, and more importantly, nursing diagnosis helps to provide a conscious and planned approach to care in an organised way. The success of nursing care is often measured by the degree of efficiency, patient satisfaction and progress.

The nursing process provides a framework that should be based on principles and roles that have been found to be highly effective in promoting quality of care. It is important to discuss the process because studies have indicated that students from often stated that they do not see evidence of the process being used in clinical practice. Even though other approaches to care may be used, such as protocols and care pathways, it is evident that the process of assessing, planning, implementation and evaluation are utilised, albeit not recorded as such.

Through the stages of the nursing process, the uniqueness and essence of nursing are explained in terms of its theoretical and scientific bases, and use of technologies and humanist suppositions that encourage critical thinking and creativity, thus improving problem solving in professional nursing practice. There is also a requirement to integrate and draw on evidence with the execution of nursing care and to examine that care critically through focused reflective practice.

PATIENT JOURNEY –
ADMISSION/TRANSFER/DISCHARGE

Emotions related to admission
All pronounced in the very young, old and mentally fragile patient.

➤ Fear of the unknown
➤ Loss of identity
➤ Disorientation
➤ Separation anxiety
➤ Loneliness
➤ Relief

A nurse's reaction to the patient can affect levels of anxiety.
Nurses should display interpersonal skills such as warmth, caring and an empathetic attitude. Show respect and maintain dignity. Adopt an individualised approach to patient care (including cultural differences) and work in collaboration with the patient.
Respect patient differences and autonomy.
Use interpreters when indicated.

Admission is the entry into a Healthcare facility.
The type of preparation and style of admission will be dependent upon whether it is:

• elective (planned)
• emergency (unplanned)
• unplanned section (mental health)

The type of transfer will be dependent upon the admission setting and the condition of the patient, e.g. from the Emergency Department, admission could be to the general/specialist wards or to the intensive care units. From a ward environment patient may be transferred to an intensive care unit or into the community (care home).

Communicate to patient and family of the transfer (where appropriate). Ensure clear documentation of the patient's condition before and during transfer to enable continuity of care.

Remember – this can be a stressful time for the patient (relocation stress).

Transfers may be internal (within the organisation) or external (outside, e.g. from one Trust to another).

Prior to admission optimise physical health.
Pre-assessment will be done for those undergoing planned admissions.

Patient may discharge themselves against medical advice.
Identify patient as high/medium/low risk.
Inform the doctor. If patient is unable to be persuaded against this, if they have capacity they should be asked to sign a self-discharge form (if still on ward).
If absconded, conduct a thorough check of the ward/environment (involve security), contact site-coordinator/police, and provide details as to what patient looks like/photo.

Complete datex form.

Demographic details

Room/bed space should be ready with the necessary equipment in place before patient arrives.

Explain hospital routine.

Give any **valuables/money** to relatives/friends to take home. If not possible then follow hospital policy for safe keeping and document.

Change patient clothing if appropriate.

Conduct an **assessment** (the timing and nature of this will be dependent upon the type of admission). Include signs and symptoms, physical, psychological, social, spiritual, cultural, risks and observations.

Formulate **plan of care**.

Discharge planning should start as soon as appropriate (as early as admission). A co-ordinated approach is required. Interprofessional meetings may be required.
Provide patient education and instructions for home care.
Information/teaching regarding medication.
Co-ordinate outpatient or home care visits. Home care assessments may need to be arranged.
If a Deprivation of Liberty Safeguard (DoLS) authorisation is required, following discharge, this should be applied for in advance.

High-risk groups:
• Older adults
• Co-morbidities
• Major surgical procedures
• Long term conditions or terminal diseases
• Learning difficulties
• Mental illness

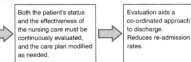

Evaluation is the last stage of the nursing process, and is an appraisal of the goal to see if it has been achieved or not.

Both the patient's status and the effectiveness of the nursing care must be continuously evaluated, and the care plan modified as needed.

Evaluation aids a co-ordinated approach to discharge. Reduces re-admission rates.

FIGURE 3.1 Admission, transfer, discharge

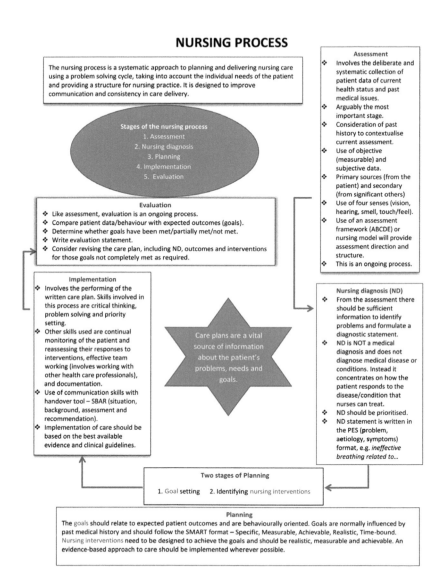

FIGURE 3.2 Nursing process

ASSESSMENT

Assessment provides the data for the identification of the patient's actual and potential health problems and needs. It also initiates the process of nursing and the basis for an individualised nursing plan and a baseline against which subsequent events can be compared. Getting to know the patient.

The assessment process also helps in establishing a rapport and developing the nurse–patient relationship, and is seen as the starting point for the partnership.

It is a dynamic and ongoing process. The assessment should be undertaken by a qualified nurse; if it is undertaken by a student nurse then this should be validated and countersigned by the qualified nurse.

Using a framework to guide assessment will help identify most (ideally all) of the patient's needs and also provide an individualised approach. Without an appropriate framework, assessment becomes meaningless.

- ABCDE assessment framework **A**irway/**B**reathing/**C**irculation/ **D**isability (neurological)/ **E**xposure (everything else) is used for the assessment of the deteriorating or acutely ill patient. It helps to quickly identify life threatening symptoms.
- Roper, Logan and Tierney Activity of Living (AL) Model Identifies 12 (AL) and includes the activity of dying. The model is used to assess the patient's dependence/independence and potential for independence in the 12 ALs.
- Orem Self-Care Model. Grounded in the belief that self-care is a fundamental requirement for effective living. Goal of nursing is to assist patient's self-care deficits. Also based on health promotion theories.
- Peplau Interpersonal Relations Model The nurse is involved in an interpersonal therapeutic relationship with the patient with the aim of reducing anxiety caused by stress through the environment or illness.
- Casey's model Designed for paediatrics and concentrates on the relationship between the health care professional and family to work in partnership. It does not provide guidance for assessment data.

Skills involved in assessment

Observation (subjective data) starts from the very first encounter with the patient. Not only of patient's physical condition but their psychological and emotional status. This can involve observing skin colour, patient's behaviour, etc.

Measuring (objective data), e.g. temperature, pulse, blood pressure, can act as a baseline.

Interviewing (subjective data) can be used to see if the non-verbal cues contradict the verbal cues. For example, a patient may say that they are not anxious, but an observation of body language could suggest otherwise.

Depending on the situation and time constraints, assessment may either be complete or focused.

Complete – provides comprehensive baseline information.

Focused – problem or need orientated. In priority order.

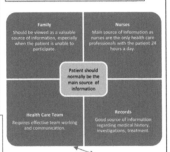

Sources of patient assessment information

History taking involves:

- ❖ biographical data (name, address, etc.)
- ❖ current physical and emotional complaints, including history of abuse (this may require skilful communication and probing, and recording in patient's own words)
- ❖ past medical and medication history
- ❖ past and current ability to perform activities of daily living
- ❖ availability of support systems
- ❖ effectiveness of past coping patterns and perceived stress
- ❖ socioeconomic factors preventing health practices
- ❖ spiritual and cultural practices/wishes/concerns.

Physical examination

Normally concentrates on the physical health complaints. Establishes a baseline.

General survey
Behaviour, demeanour.

Inspection
Taking and recording vital signs (guidelines exist for the paediatric environments). Observe for colour, size, location, movement, texture, symmetry, odours, sounds. Use relevant assessment tools, e.g. pain tool.

Diagnostic testing data

Blood profiles, X-rays, CT scans, endoscopies etc.

Nurse should ensure that the patient is safely and appropriately prepared, and monitor for post complications. They should also be able to access results.

Data should be collected and organised in a methodical and structured way. It should also be guided by the documentation in use in the practice setting at the time of assessment.

Documentation should follow the principles of the Code (NMC 2018b).

FIGURE 3.3 Assessment

PLANNING

There are two main stages here: 1. Identification of goals, 2. Identification of appropriate nursing interventions to achieve these goals. Goal statements (or expected patient outcomes) are formulated after reviewing the assessment data and problems/nursing diagnostic statements have been formulated. A nursing diagnosis may require more than one expected patient outcome.

Goal statements provide information regarding what nursing is aiming to achieve in relation to the patient problems and how these aims will be met. By producing a comprehensive plan of care the scope of nursing responsibilities is acknowledged, as are those specific actions for which nurses are prepared to hold themselves accountable.

This should be patient oriented and involve the patient. Helping patients to assume greater responsibility for their own health is an important focus of activity for all nurses and helps maximise patient compliance.

Goals should be written in relation to the patient's observable behaviour (performance) and not nursing actions. Therefore goals should be positive statements and measurable.
Goals should contain the following elements:
1. **Who** is to demonstrate the desired behaviour, i.e. *the patient*.
2. The **desired behaviour** that will demonstrate the goal has been achieved, *e.g. will drink*.
3. The **measurement** that will be used to evaluate the behaviour, to assess success, *e.g. 2.5 litres of fluid*.
4. The **relevant conditions** under which the behaviour will be performed, *e.g. fluid of patient's choice*.
5. By what **time** it is expected that the behaviour will be achieved. This will be dependent upon the urgency of the problem (may be immediate or longer-term), *e.g. 24 hours*.

Example: The patient will drink 2.5 litres of fluid of their choice in 24 hours.

Broad aims of care can be written and give direction to specific goals identified for patients, which can themselves be regarded as steps on the way to more general, ultimate desirable outcomes. If written as broad aims, this direction may become meaningless (e.g. a patient should 'maintain maximum independence'). Instead, aims should be broken down to specific goals where possible.

Some goals may not have a specific time span because they are there as a source of direction where it is hard to attach a specific attainment date.

Short-term goals

Some of these goals require immediate action as in an emergency situation, but most are goals that need to be achieved within a 48-hour period (e.g. drink 2.5 litres of fluid in 24 hours).

Medium-term goals

These may not be considered but should have the time frame of approximately one to four weeks.

Long-term goals

Have much longer time spans, usually two weeks to one month.

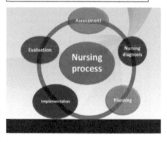

Interventions

These can be either **independent** (falls within the scope of nursing practice only) or **collaborative** (involvement of interprofessional team). Interventions should:

➢ be based on the identified goals
➢ be based on existing credible evidence
➢ be comprehensive enough to ensure that the patient can meet the outcomes
➢ always begin with an action verb (e.g. monitor, offer, discuss)
➢ be kept simple and to the point
➢ clearly state the necessary action
➢ be suited to the patient concerned
➢ be safe and produce no harm
➢ adhere to policies and procedures in place
➢ be based on evidence-based practice
➢ consider other health care activities
➢ use available resources.

Professional knowledge is necessary to identify the appropriate behaviour which should be indicative of the goal being set. The appropriate level of goal will be dependent upon the assessment data.
Goals should be **SMART**:
   Specific
   Measurable
   Achievable
   Realistic
   Time-bound

FIGURE 3.4 Planning

IMPLEMENTATION

This stage involves the application of the nursing care plan. This means 'hands on' involvement. Implementation entails:

- Employing planned interventions
- Using critical thinking skills
- Problem solving
- Setting priorities
- Continuous reassessment of patients' responses to the interventions
- Effective team working and communication
- Documentation

Types of interventions will be dependent upon the patients set goals, but may include:

- ❖ Assessment and monitoring
- ❖ Administration of medicines
- ❖ Collecting specimens
- ❖ Offering comfort measures
- ❖ Providing nourishment and fluids
- ❖ Helping with Activities of Daily Living (ADL)
- ❖ Supporting body functions, e.g. respiration (oxygen therapy), hydration (IV fluids)
- ❖ Providing hygiene and skin care
- ❖ Offering emotional support
- ❖ Offering spiritual support
- ❖ Providing teaching and counselling

Organisation of work

Putting an individualised plan of care into action demands organisational skill and every new care plan presents a new organisational challenge.

Systems of work organisation can be through the following:

Task allocation – care is broken down into a series of tasks, e.g. administration of medicines, observations, patient washes, and are normally hierarchical in nature. Here, nurses have a brief encounter with a large number of patients. Each patient encounters many different nurses.

Patient allocation – each nurse is delegated responsibility for the care of a group of patients for the duration of a shift. This approach can deteriorate to task allocation.

Primary nursing – one nurse assumes the total nursing care and co-ordination of a group of 3–6 patients from admission to discharge. They are accountable for this care, which does not cease when they are off duty – they work with an associate who delivers care according to the plan when the primary nurse is absent.

Sources of information about the patient can be found from:

- listening to the handover at each shift change
- reading patient observation charts, care plans, medical notes
- talking to the patients themselves, family members, other staff
- directly observing and assessing the patients
- reviewing laboratory and other test results.

Implementation

In order to maximise effectiveness and efficiency and promote patient rest, try to integrate as many interventions in one visit as is possible. This not only helps you gain a more holistic picture of the patient, but will also help with time management.

Co-ordination and integration of nursing care between or with ADL, medication administration, observations, treatments and other collaborative and interdependent care have several benefits:

- ➢ Saves time
- ➢ Enhances co-ordination and management skills
- ➢ Allows the provision of efficient and timely care
- ➢ Allows patient time to rest

Nurses must develop and maintain a therapeutic working relationship with patients in order to establish an efficient and effective nurse–patient partnership and work towards a common goal. With the child this will be a partnership with the family/parents.

Partnership involves an individualised and personal approach to care, sharing knowledge, information and the performing of care. The power relationship should be equal. There should be a strong element of trust brought into the relationship so that it is positive and becomes a helping relationship with mutual respect.

Through the implementation of care there are ample opportunities to listen to the patient (either through their verbal or non-verbal communication, i.e. messages that are transmitted without using words, e.g. facial expressions, gestures). Remember non-verbal cues may contradict what is said verbally. Actions speak greater than words.

Therapeutic use of touch can convey warmth and understanding but needs to be used sensitively. Inappropriate invasion of personal space can be discomforting or even irritating by the recipient.

Establish boundaries of the relationship and, where/when appropriate, increase patient level of autonomy (if not established). This is particularly pertinent in a mental health setting – do not enforce dependency.

FIGURE 3.5 Implementation

EVALUATION

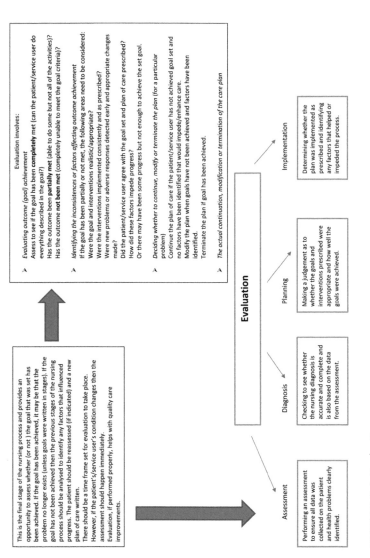

This is the final stage of the nursing process and provides an opportunity to assess whether (or not) the goal that was set has been achieved. If the goal has been achieved, it may be that the problem no longer exists (unless goals were written in stages). If the goal has not been achieved then the previous stages of the nursing process should be analysed to identify any factors that influenced progress. The patient should be reassessed (if indicated) and a new plan of care written.

There should be a time frame set for evaluation to take place.

However, if the patient's/service user's condition changes then the assessment should happen immediately.

Evaluation, if performed properly, helps with quality care improvements.

Evaluation involves:

➢ *Evaluating outcome (goal) achievement*
Assess to see if the goal has been **completely met** (can the patient/service user do everything described in the goal?)
Has the outcome been **partially met** (able to do some but not all of the activities)?
Has the outcome **not been met** (completely unable to meet the goal criteria)?

➢ *Identifying the inconsistencies or factors affecting outcome achievement*
If the goal has been partially or not met, the following areas need to be considered:
Were the goal and interventions realistic/appropriate?
Were the interventions implemented consistently and as prescribed?
Were new problems or adverse responses detected early and appropriate changes made?
Did the patient/service user agree with the goal set and plan of care prescribed?
How did these factors impede progress?
Or there may have been some progress but not enough to achieve the set goal.

➢ *Deciding whether to continue, modify or terminate the plan (for a particular problem)*
Continue the plan of care if the patient/service user has not achieved goal set and no factors have been identified that would impede/enhance care.
Modify the plan when goals have not been achieved and factors have been identified.
Terminate the plan if goal has been achieved.

➢ *The actual continuation, modification or termination of the care plan*

Evaluation

Assessment

Performing an assessment to ensure all data was collected on the patient and health problems clearly identified.

Diagnosis

Checking to see whether the nursing diagnosis is accurate and complete and is also based on the data from the assessment.

Planning

Making a judgement as to whether the goals and interventions prescribed were appropriate and how well the goals were achieved.

Implementation

Determining whether the plan was implemented as prescribed and identifying any factors that helped or impeded the process.

FIGURE 3.6 Evaluation

Activity: now test yourself

1   The stages of the nursing process are:

    a   Assessment, evaluation, implementation, planning, diagnosis

    b   Evaluation, implementation, planning, assessment, diagnosis

    c   Assessment, implementation, planning, diagnosis, evaluation

    d   Assessment, diagnosis, planning, implementation, evaluation

2   State whether true or false:

    a   Care can be provided to the patient without the first stage of the nursing process

    b   Evaluation is the large stage and the patient/service user's outcomes are compared with the goal set

    c   Planning consists of two stages: goal setting and pre-scribing nursing care

3   List four emotions that can be associated with admission to hospital

4   When caring for a patient/client, where would you get information from to help you care for this person appropriately

Answers

1 d
The nursing process is an organised, systematic approach to the management of patient care that consists of five sequential and interrelated stages. These stages are: assessment, diagnosis, planning, implementation and evaluation. As one stage informs the next stage, if used out of sequence, quality of care would be compromised and potentially harmful to patients because inappropriate care may be delivered to the patient/service user

2 a False
Assessment is arguably the most important stage because it provides information/data that will affect the other stages and the provision of nursing care

   b True

   c True

3 Any four of the following:

   Fear of the unknown
   Loss of identity
   Disorientation
   Separation anxiety
   Loneliness
   Relief

4 Any from the following list (you may have more to add):

   Listening to the handover/conversations about the patient/ service user
   Reading patient observation charts, care plans, medical notes
   Talking to the patient themselves, family members, other staff
   Directly observing and assessing the patient
   Reviewing laboratory and other test results

Reflection: ask yourself

1 What do I know that I did not know before?

2 What I am confused about now?

3 What areas do I need to focus on?

4 My action plan for further learning (make objectives SMART)

CHAPTER 4

End-of-life care

Sheila Cunningham

Overview

End-of-life care is support for people who are in the last months or years of their life. People who are approaching the end of their life are entitled to high-quality care, wherever they are being cared for.

Link to *Future Nurse Proficiencies* (NMC 2018a)

Platform 3 Assessing needs and planning care: specifically 3.14
Platform 4 Planning and evaluating care: specifically 4.9
Annexe B: Nursing procedures Section 10: use evidence-based, best practice approaches for meeting needs for care and support at the end of life, accurately assessing the person's capacity for independence and self-care, and initiating appropriate interventions

Expected knowledge

- Lifespan and causes of dying
- Comfort measures for patients

Introduction

End-of-life care is a feature within many areas: medical wards, emergency rooms and intensive care, in fact in all places where patients are cared for. This points to the need for nurses and all care workers in any area to be able to deliver high-quality end-of-life care. End-of-life is provided by a range of organisations; within the NHS provision, patients may be admitted to general medical or oncology wards or receive care in the community from district nurses, health visitors or specialist community end-of-life-care nurses. Within the community this applies to people of all ages ethnicities, beliefs, and social and personal circumstances. It is a challenge and requires a real reflection on a professional's value base, focus on person-centred care and their woes, and acknowledgement that it is loaded with emotion for all concerned.

Content

End-of-life care priorities	Symptom assessment and management	Care of the body after death
Spiritual care	End-of-life care in specific groups	Ethical issues

Learning outcomes

- Define end-of-life care
- Use evidence-based, best practice approaches for meeting needs for care and support at the end of life, accurately assessing the person's capacity for independence and self-care
- Identify issues with symptom control and the interventions available to address these issues
- Identify interventions appropriate for a range of patients in a diverse range of settings at the end of their life
- Explain and justify the procedures before and after the episode of death

Key background

Nurses will inevitably come across people in a variety of setting who may have life-limiting disorders. It is important, therefore, for nurses to be aware of needs of people and families for care at the end of life, whether this is for short or prolonged periods of end-of-life care. The NHS (2017) indicates that end-of-life care should enable patients to live as well as possible until they die and then to die with dignity. Furthermore, each patient has the right to express their wishes about where they would like to receive care and where they would like to die. This may be challenging and create stress for patients and their loved ones, depending on their needs towards their final days. End-of-life care is offered in their own homes, care homes, hospices or hospitals, depending on their needs or preferences. What is important to people and their families must be prioritised when providing evidence-based, person-centred nursing care at the end of life, including the care of people who are dying, families, the deceased and the bereaved. The terms 'end-of-life care' and 'palliative care' are often used interchangeably, but are different. *Palliative care* is the treatment, care and support of people with a life-limiting illness, and their family and friends. It is sometimes called 'supportive care'. This does not mean that patients are at the end of life, but can be given at any point during illnesses, for any period of time, and sometimes parallel with other treatments, therapies and medicines aimed at controlling their illness, such as chemotherapy or radiotherapy. *End-of-life care* involves the treatment, care and support for people who are nearing the end of their life and is an important part of palliative care. Nurses must therefore be conscious of this, and their role in identifying and assessing the needs of patients with a life-limiting disorder, including requirements for palliative care and decision-making related to their treatment and care preferences.

PRIORITIES FOR CARE OF THE DYING PERSON

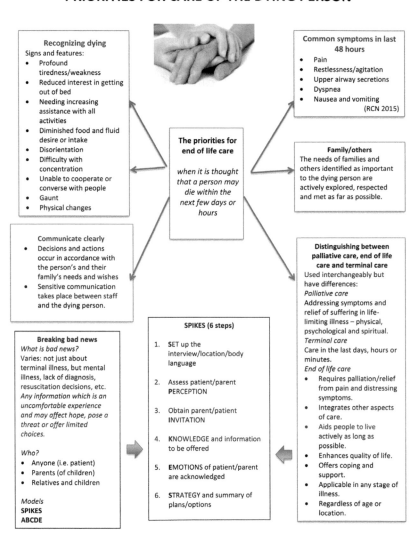

Recognizing dying
Signs and features:
- Profound tiredness/weakness
- Reduced interest in getting out of bed
- Needing increasing assistance with all activities
- Diminished food and fluid desire or intake
- Disorientation
- Difficulty with concentration
- Unable to cooperate or converse with people
- Gaunt
- Physical changes

Common symptoms in last 48 hours
- Pain
- Restlessness/agitation
- Upper airway secretions
- Dyspnea
- Nausea and vomiting
(RCN 2015)

The priorities for end of life care

when it is thought that a person may die within the next few days or hours

Family/others
The needs of families and others identified as important to the dying person are actively explored, respected and met as far as possible.

Communicate clearly
- Decisions and actions occur in accordance with the person's and their family's needs and wishes
- Sensitive communication takes place between staff and the dying person.

Distinguishing between palliative care, end of life care and terminal care
Used interchangeably but have differences:
Palliative care
Addressing symptoms and relief of suffering in life-limiting illness – physical, psychological and spiritual.
Terminal care
Care in the last days, hours or minutes.
End of life care
- Requires palliation/relief from pain and distressing symptoms.
- Integrates other aspects of care.
- Aids people to live actively as long as possible.
- Enhances quality of life.
- Offers coping and support.
- Applicable in any stage of illness.
- Regardless of age or location.

Breaking bad news
What is bad news?
Varies: not just about terminal illness, but mental illness, lack of diagnosis, resuscitation decisions, etc. *Any information which is an uncomfortable experience and may affect hope, pose a threat or offer limited choices.*

Who?
- Anyone (i.e. patient)
- Parents (of children)
- Relatives and children

Models
SPIKES
ABCDE

SPIKES (6 steps)

1. **S**ET up the interview/location/body language

2. Assess patient/parent **P**ERCEPTION

3. Obtain parent/patient **I**NVITATION

4. **K**NOWLEDGE and information to be offered

5. **E**MOTIONS of patient/parent are acknowledged

6. **S**TRATEGY and summary of plans/options

FIGURE 4.1 Priorities in end-of-life care

CARE OF PERSON AFTER DEATH

Care of the body after death

The nurse or health care professional records (notes) the time, who was present, the nature of the death, and details of any relevant devices (such as cardiac defibrillators) and calls the doctor.

The identity of the deceased is verified by a doctor to certify death (document).

Ensure relatives are informed and offer support (significant others, religious or spiritual contact).

Physical tasks: as soon as possible

- Lay the deceased flat (while supporting the head with a pillow) and preparing them and the room for viewing.
- Family viewing/spending time with the deceased. Offer age-appropriate support (e.g. for children).
- Pack and document personal property showing consideration for the feelings of those receiving it (local policy).
- Discuss the issue of soiled clothes sensitively with the family (disposed of or returned).

Preparation and respect

- Be calm, respectful and treat the deceased as a person who was living until recently.
- Within some religions, last offices may be performed by a member of the religion.
- Note: cares should be carried out with due regard to infection control and manual handling policies.

Personal care of the body after death position

1. Lay the deceased person on their back, limbs straight (if possible), arms by their sides.
2. A pillow under the head supports the body and helps the mouth stay closed (or use a rolled towel).
3. Close the eyes by applying light pressure.

Coroner?

Check local policy – if sudden death does Coroner need to be informed?

Guides and informs personal care practices.

Physical cares

1. Comb or tidy the deceased's hair.
2. IF no coroner involved: remove mechanical aids, such as syringe drivers, apply gauze and tape to syringe driver sites and document disposal of medication.
3. Leakage may occur: cover wounds, stomas, lines, padding for bladder or bowels.
4. Wash the deceased (unless requested or prohibited by faith or culture), maintaining dignity throughout.
5. Dress the deceased in the appropriate clothing (in hospital possibly a shroud; in a community setting it may be their own clothes).

Transfer

1. Check the deceased has identity and this is securely fastened onto the body.
2. Gently wrap the deceased in a clean sheet and secure loosely.
3. Transfer the body to the mortuary (in hospital) or in community setting this may be to the undertaker.
4. At all times be respectful and sensitive.

FIGURE 4.2 Care of the body after death

SPIRITUAL CARE AND RELIGIOUS CONSIDERATIONS FOR DYING PERSON AND FAMILY

Spiritual care

Spirituality means different things to different people. Religion and faith might be part of someone's spirituality, but spirituality is not always religious. Spiritual needs can include:

- the need for meaning and purpose in their lives
- the need to love and feel loved
- the need for a sense of belonging
- the need to feel hope, peace and gratitude.

People do different things to meet these spiritual needs, depending on what's important to them. This may change over the course of a lifetime.

Spirituality – is it religion?

There is a general lack of clarity with regard to the meanings of the terms 'spirituality', 'religion' and, indeed, 'well-being'. Spirituality is summarised as: the way in which people understand and live their lives in view of their core beliefs and values and their perception of ultimate meaning.
(Holloway *et al.* 2009)

Spiritual assessment tool

There are several, but the following are useful:

FICA

An acronym that can be used to remember what is asked in a spiritual history is:

- Faith or Beliefs
- Importance and influence
- Community
- Address

The HOPE spiritual assessment

Hope, sources of hope, meaning, comfort strength, peace, love, connection
Organised religion
Personal practices
Effects on medical care and end of life issues.
(Old and Swaggerty 2007)

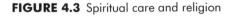

Skills for spiritual care

- Techniques of active and compassionate listening
- Companioning
- Non-denominational spiritual practices, such as prayer, contemplation and meditation
- Specialist chaplaincy skills and services to fulfil religious needs or practices

Resources

To aid in supporting people with religious beliefs at the point of dying include:

Association of Hospice and Palliative care Chaplains: Multifaith guide
http://www.ahpcc.org.uk/practical-resources/multi_faith-chaplaincy-resources/

Marie Curie Hospices: Faith
https://www.mariecurie.org.uk/profesionals/palliative-care-knowledge-zone

Religions to be aware of

Data collected from the 2011 Census highlighted that the six biggest religions in England and Wales are Christianity, Islam, Hinduism, Sikhism, Judaism and Buddhism in order of population size.
(PHE 2016)

Changes to religious affinity include:

- Reduced number or people identifying with Christianity.
- Increase in people identifying with other religions, specifically Islam (2.7 million people).
- Next are identifying affinity to the following: Hindu; Sikh; Judaism and Buddhism.
(ONS 2012)

FIGURE 4.3 Spiritual care and religion

ETHICAL ISSUES AND CHALLENGES IN END OF LIFE CARE

Ethical dilemmas
There is a range of key ethical issues and dilemmas debated in EoLC.

Do not resuscitate orders:
- Withdrawal of feeding and hydration
- Advance directives
- Assisted suicide
- Euthanasia

Key considerations:
Debate openly and honestly – clarify misunderstandings or confusion.
Share decision making (family and care team).
Empower people and recognise emotional challenges.

Advance decision and advance statement?

An advance statement is a written statement that sets out persons preferences, wishes, beliefs and values regarding the future care (NHS 2017):

- Not legally binding
- Do not need to be witnessed

It is a useful communication and preparation, and is open to change and amendment.

Consent and advance decision

An **advance decision** (sometimes known as an advance decision to refuse treatment, an ADRT, or a living will) is a decision a person makes to refuse a specific type of treatment at some time in the future.
Addressed in the *Mental Capacity Act* (2019), concerning consent and adults over 18 years.

It needs to be clear in addressing:
- Refusing which treatment in what specific situations, but not others.
- Indicating all the circumstances in which the person refuses treatment.

Conditions for advance decision (or advance decision to refuse treatment) include:
- Person has mental capacity and competence to make the decision
- It is a fully informed decision and the consequences are clear
- The person states the advance directive applies to all circumstances
- No one has influenced or pressured the person making this decision
(NHS 2017)

Children and dying

Child dying
Complex care and parental involvement.
Involves complex decisions and advance care planning for symptom control and management.
Caring for children of dying adults (parents etc.)
Also challenging. Care includes:
- Information: honest and age appropriate
- Space: to share and express feelings
- Routine: for sense of safety
- A key person: for support and continuity
- Connection: to the dying person through building mementos etc.
- Support in bereavement, perhaps specialist bereavement services.

Homelessness and end of life care
St Mungos and Marie Curie (2017) provide resources to address this.

They suggest these key issues are considered for the homeless person:

- Identifying who are the key supporting people at the end stage of life
- Asking residents/persons to devise an eco-map of people important to them in their lives
- Hostel or other accommodation support: resources and personnel
- Offering support and palliation acceptable to the dying person

What can be refused?

Treatment that replaces or supports ailing bodily functions, such as:
- Ventilation – to aid breathing
- Cardiopulmonary resuscitation (CPR)
- Antibiotics – for infections

FIGURE 4.4 Ethical challenges in end-of-life care

Activity: now test yourself

1 What does S in SPIKES stand for?

  a sitting down

  b standing up

  c setting the scene

  d space

2 Advance care planning is planning for what a person may or may not want at the very end of life, and can be done at any stage as long as the person has capacity.

  a True

  b False

3 Documentation is useful to aid communication between teams:

  a True

  b False

4 Providing open and honest information about impending death can help a person in bereavement.

  a True

  b False

5 Which of the following are physical changes that may be apparent 1–2 weeks before dying?

  a Decreased blood pressure

  b Increased perspiration

  c Agitation

  d Congestion

  e All of the above

Answers

1 c   Setting the scene
   Recall: scene setting, perception, invitation, knowledge, empathy, summary

2 a   True
   This is not legally binding or need to be witnessed, but is a communication route for sharing a dying person's wishes and needs.

3 a   True
   For the same reason as above – information is best written down so that it can be shared and is clear. Teams change and the same person is not necessarily at every meeting or available.

4 a   True
   Relatives and loved ones, even children, appreciate open and honest conversations. They cannot predict death and, given that bereavement starts before death, the process of and opportunity to say farewell and share memories, and anything they wish, or even to prepare themselves emotionally or psychologically, can be realised.

5 e   All of the above
   As physical processes decline, physiological changes occur to all the organs and processes – features include alterations in homeostasis, and the usual functions such as bladder and bowel functions. Disease processes or medications may also intensify these.

Reflection: ask yourself

1   What do I know now that I didn't know before?

2   What am I confused/unclear about?

3   What areas do I need to focus on?

4   My action plan for further learning (make objectives SMART)

Bibliography

Alzheimer's Society (2017) *What not to say to somebody with dementia* (online). Available at: www.alzheimers.org.uk/blog/language-dementia-what-not-to-say (accessed 22 May 2019).

Bunch, C. (2017) *Manual for Caldicott Guardians*. London: UK Caldicott Guardian Council. Available from https://assets.publishing.service.gov.uk/government/uploads/system/uploads/attachment_data/file/581213/cgmanual.pdf (accessed 11 November 2019).

Department of Health (2003) *Confidentiality: NHS Code of Practice*. London. Department of Health.

Data Protection Act (1998) London: HMSO. Available at: www.legislation.gov.uk/ukpga/1998/29/contents (accessed 11 November 2019).

Department of Health (2012) *Compassion in Practice: Nursing, midwifery and care staff, our vision and strategy*. London: Department of Health.

Egan, G. (2010) *The Skilled Helper: A problem management and opportunity development approach to helping*. 9th edition. Pacific Grove, CA: Brooks/Cole.

Francis, R. (2013) *Report of the Mid Staffordshire NHS Foundation Trust Public Inquiry*, vol. 3. *Present and Future Annexes*. London: The Stationery Office.

Freedom of Information Act (1998) London: HMSO. Available at: www.legislation.gov.uk/ukpga/2000/36/contents (accessed 11 November 2019).

Holloway, M., Adamson, S., McSherry, W. and Swinton. J. (2009) *Spiritual Care at the End of Life: A systematic review of the literature*. London: Department of Health.

Huston, C.J. (2014) *Professional Issues in Nursing: Challenges & opportunities*, 3rd edn. Philadelphia, PA: Wolters Kluwer/Lippincott, Williams & Wilkins.

Keogh, B. (2013) *Review into the Quality of Care and Treatment Provided by 14 Hospital Trusts in England: Overview Report*. London: NHS.

Marie Curie (2018) *What are palliative care and end of life care?* Available at: www.mariecurie.org.uk/help/support/diagnosed/recent-diagnosis/palliative-care-end-of-life-care (accessed 6 January 2018).

Mental Capacity (Amendment) Act (2019) London: HMSO. Available at: www.legislation.gov.uk/ukpga/2019/18/enacted (accessed 11 November 2019).

Murdoch, H. (2009) *A Curriculum for Multi-sensory-impaired Children from MSI Unit Victoria School Birmingham*. London: Sense.

National Health Service (NHS) (2017) End of life care (online). Available at: www.nhs.uk/conditions/end-of-life-care/advance-statement (accessed 20 May 2019).

National Institute for Health and Care Excellence (NICE) (2017a) *Care of Dying Adults in the Last Days of Life: Quality standard [QS144].* London: NICE Available at: www.nice.org.uk/guidance/qs144 (accessed 6 January 2018).

National Institute for Health and Care Excellence (NICE) (2017b) *End of Life Care for Infants, Children and Young People: Quality standard [QS160].* London: NICE. Available at: www.nice.org.uk/guidance/qs160 (accessed 6 January 2018).

National Council of State Boards (1995) *Delegation: Concepts and decision-making process.* Wellington: National Council of State Boards.

Nursing and Midwifery Council (NMC) (2018a) *Future Nurse Proficiencies.* London: NMC. Available at: www.nmc.org.uk/standards/standards-for-nurses/standards-of-proficiency-for-registered-nurses (accessed 1 May 19).

Nursing and Midwifery Council (NMC) (2018b) *The Code: Professional standards of practice and behaviour.* London: NMC.

Nursing and Midwifery Council (NMC) (2018c) *Delegation and Account-ability: Supplementary information to the Code.* London: NMC.

Nursing and Midwifery Council (NMC) (2019a) *Revalidation: How to revalidate with the NMC.* London: NMC.

Nursing and Midwifery Council (NMC) (2019b) *Guidance on the Profes-sional Duty of Candour.* London: NMC.

Office for National Statistics (ONS) (2012) *Full Story: What does the Census tell us about religion in 2011?* London: ONS. Available at: www.ons.gov.uk/peoplepopulationandcommunity/culturalidentity/religion/articles/fullstorywhatdoesthecensustellusaboutreligionin 2011/2013-05-16 (accessed 1 May 2019).

Old, J.L and Swaggerty, D.L. (2007) *A Practical Guide to Palliative Care.* Philadelphia, PA: Lippincott, Williams and Wilkins.

Public Health England (PHE) (2016) *Faith at End of Life: A resource for professionals, providers and commissioners working in communities.* London: Public Health England.

Royal College of Nursing (RCN) (2017a) *Standards for Assessing, Measuring and Monitoring Vital Signs in Infants, Children and Young People.* London: RCN.

Public Records Act (1958) London: HMSO. Available at: www.legislation.gov.uk/ukpga/Eliz2/6-7/51 (accessed 11 November 2019).

Royal College of Nursing (RCN) (2010) *Principles of Nursing Practice.* London: RCN.

Royal College of Nursing (RCN) (2015) *Getting it Right Every Time: Funda-mentals of nursing care at the end of life.* Available at http://rcnendoflife.org.uk/symptom-management/ (accessed 11 November 2019).

Royal College of Nursing (RCN) (2017b) *Accountability and Delegation.* London: RCN.

Royal College of Nursing (RCN) (2019) *Revalidation.* London: RCN.

St Mungo's and Marie Curie (2017) *Palliative Care* (online). Available at: www.mungos.org/service_model/palliative-care (accessed 21 May 2019).

Index

Page numbers in *italics* denote figures.

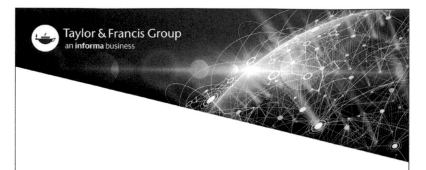